SJÖGREN'S SYNDROME GUIDE

A Personal Survival Journey through Sjögren's Syndrome (Navigating the Silent Storm)

Clattern A. Risant

Table of Contents

Chapter One

Introduction

Sjögren's syndrome is a chronic autoimmune disease characterized by eyes and mouth dryness resulting from lacrimal and salivary gland dysfunction. As a result, the disease is characterized by pleomorphic clinical manifestations whose characteristics and severity may differ largely from one patient to another.

The actual causes of sjögren's syndrome are still unknown. Nevertheless, different, not mutually exclusive, models involving genetic and environmental factors have been put forward to explain its development. The emergence of aberrant autoreactive B-lymphocytes, conducting autoantibody production and immune complex formation, seems crucial in developing the disease. It is challenging to diagnose Sjögren's syndrome because there is a variation in the signs and symptoms in different individuals, which may resemble those of other diseases.

Sjögren's syndrome is a chronic autoimmune condition that occurs when the immune system attacks the glands that produce moisture in the eyes, mouth, and other body parts. The primary symptoms are dry eyes and mouth; other parts of the body may be affected, and many people complain of joint and muscle pain with fatigue. The severe stage of sjögren's syndrome can lead to damage to the lungs, kidneys and nervous system. Sjögren's syndrome can occur alone or with other autoimmune disorders, for example, rheumatoid arthritis or systemic lupus erythematosus.

Presently, there is no known cure for Sjögren's syndrome, but different ways of management and treatment of the symptoms exist.

Women are mostly affected by Sjögren's syndrome. There is no age limit at which one can have Sjögren's syndrome, but it is most common in people ages 40 and 50. It has no geographical boundary, as it affects all ethnic and racial groups.

There are two forms of Sjögren's syndrome:

- Primary form: People who have this type are those who do not have other rheumatic diseases.

- Secondary form: People who have this type are those who have other rheumatic diseases, for example, rheumatoid arthritis, systemic lupus erythematosus, and scleroderma.

At 42, I experienced dry eyes, thinking that longer hours on the computer may have caused it. Then around 50, I developed a very dry mouth as well. At this time, I was working hard to establish a new company based on technology transfer.

In August 2018 I started experiencing symptoms of what the doctor diagnosed as lupus, including the classic eye-mask rash, and shoulder pain.

It took almost a year to get a diagnosis of lupus with central nervous system involvement and Sjögren's syndrome. My family doesn't have a strong history of autoimmune disease, although my brother had severe eczema and asthma. Now I know autoimmune diseases are highly connected to each other.

Besides the several immunosuppressants I'm taking right now for lupus, I am also dependent on two types of eye drops, special toothpaste and a mouth spray to maintain good oral health.

One big challenge with autoimmune disease is that the continuous attacks on the organs will lead to irreparable damage over time, so the earlier you get diagnosed and deal with the peaks of inflammation the better.

This book was produced with the sole aim of providing a comprehensive guide for managing and coping with sjögren's syndrome.

Chapter Two

Understanding Sjögren's Syndrome

Sjögren syndrome is identified as an autoimmune condition, one among many health conditions which occur as a result of the immune system attacking the body's own tissues and organs. What happens in sjögren's syndrome is that the immune system targets the glands that produce tears (lacrimal glands) and saliva (salivary glands), reducing the glands' ability to produce these fluids.

Dry eyes can result in burning, itching and that feeling of the presence of sand in your eyes, inability to focus on bright or fluorescent lighting. When your mouth is dry, you can feel as if there are particles of chalk in your mouth, and persons affected may experience difficulty speaking, swallowing, or tasting food.

The situation in which the immune system attacks and damages other organs and tissues are known as extra glandular involvement.

Those affected experience swelling in connective tissues, which gives flexibility and strength to structures around the body. Conditions that involve swelling of connective tissue are most times referred to as rheumatic disorders. In Sjögren's syndrome, extra glandular involvement may lead to painful swelling of the joints and muscles; dry, itchy skin and skin rashes; persistent cough; a hoarse voice; kidney and liver conditions; numbness and tingling sensation in the hands and feet; and, in most women, vaginal dryness. Continuous tiredness (fatigue) is severe enough to hinder daily activities. Other autoimmune conditions can also occur after the emergence of sjögren's syndrome.

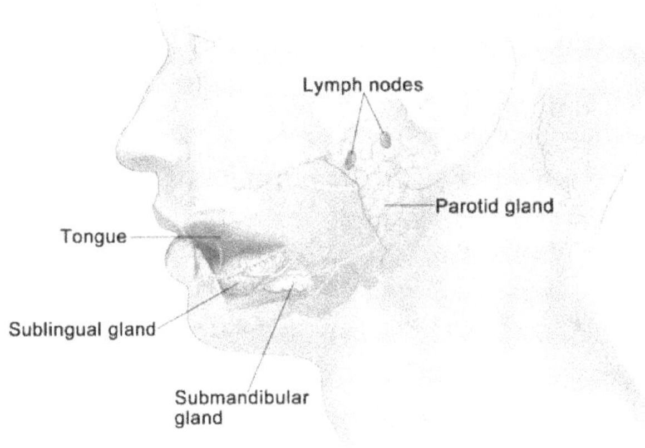

The Origin of Sjögren's Syndrome

The idiom Sjögren's disease was derived from a Swedish ophthalmologist by the name of Henrik Sjögren (1899 – 1986). He was the first person who identified a group of women and correlated the triad of keratoconjuctiva sicca, xerostomia and polyarthritis. He was a graduate of Medicine from Karolinska Institute in 1918 and qualified as a physician in 1927. His interest in ophthalmology started as early as 1925 when he identified the first patient's classical symptoms which were to bear his name and whose name bears the title. His continuous interest in ophthalmology led him to establish the first department of ophthalmology in a Swedish town where his interest in corneal grafting was developed.

The first reported case of dry eyes and mouth was demonstrated by both J.W. Hutchinson and W.B. Hadden. Sjögren's syndrome is similar to Sicca complex syndrome and Mikulicz's disease. "Sicca" is a Latin word which means dryness and was used together with keratoconjunctivitis to derive the word "keratoconjunctivitis sicca" explaining the dryness of the cornea and conjunctiva.

Mikulicz disease got its name in 1888, through von Mikulicz Radecki which is a sub-set of Sjögren's disease and shows the enlargement of the parotid, submandibular and lacrimal glands.

There were also further reports of these classical symptoms by a Frenchman in 1925 by name Gougerot's syndrome which also identified the three classical symptoms of dry eyes, dry mouth and polyarthritis.

At first, when Henrik Sjögren published his book, this was unnoticed and he was not given the title of docent and his academic role as an ophthalmologist was hindered.

His work was later published in English in the year 1943 and at this period he was given recognition for his work and was awarded the position of an associate professor at the University of Gothenburg and was honoured with the title of professor in 1961.

It is not enough that Henrik Sjögren was the first person to correlate the triad of keratoconjuctiva sicca, xerostomia and polyarthritis but he provided the ground for defining this condition by his title and the name of all his predecessors were superseded.

Henrik Sjögren died on the 17th September 1986. His expertise not only led to the definition of Sjögren disease but he was also the first person to develop the recognition of corneal grafting. He used his expertise in different specialties for which he was honoured with a position in the ophthalmological society of Australia and the American rheumatism board.

Causes of Sjögren's Syndrome

Presently, there is no actual cause of sjögren's syndrome. These factors may play a role:

- Environmental factors.

- Genetics.

- Viral infections.

An environmental factor may change the immune system and result in immune damage later on, such as infection with hepatitis C or the Epstein-Barr virus. As women are mostly affected by sjögren's, a theory has it that estrogen, a female hormone, plays a vital role. However, this has not been proven.

As I earlier stated in the introductory part of this book, there are two forms of sjögren's syndrome: the primary form and the secondary form. The causes of Sjögren's Syndrome will be discussed under these two forms.

Causes of Primary Sjögren's Syndrome

Primary Sjögren's syndrome is an autoimmune disorder which presents dry eyes (keratoconjunctivitis sicca) and dry mouth (xerostomia) as a result of infiltration of lymphocytic lacrimal and salivary glands. Primary Sjögren's syndrome does not occur with another autoimmune condition. Primary Sjögren's syndrome can be caused by a medical condition, environmental factors, medications, and even lifestyle choices.

Causes of Secondary Sjögren's Syndrome

Secondary Sjögren's syndrome exists with any other autoimmune condition, such as Hepatitis C, IgG4 Disease, polymyositis, Rheumatoid Arthritis (RA), Scleroderma, and Systemic Lupus Erythematosus. Secondary Sjögren's syndrome is identified when someone with an existing autoimmune disease, such as scleroderma or lupus, experiences dry eyes and mouth.

Symptoms of Sjögren's syndrome

The primary symptoms of sjögren's syndrome are dry eyes and mouth, some persons complain of joint and muscle pains all over their bodies, and I experienced similar things during my episode. Other symptoms include:

- Dry cough or hoarseness.

- Fatigue.

- Blurry vision.

- Abnormal sense of taste.

- Enlargement of salivary glands.

- Burning or redness in eyes, or grittiness (like sand).

- Difficulty chewing, swallowing or talking.

- Dry, itchy skin.

- Tiredness

- Rashes (mostly after exposure to sunlight)

- Vaginal dryness

Manifestations of Sjögren's Syndrome

Oral dryness can profoundly affect the quality of life, interfering with basic daily functions such as eating, speaking, and sleeping. Low secretion of tears may lead to chronic irritation and destruction of corneal and bulbar conjunctival epithelium (keratoconjunctivitis sicca).

Mucous gland secretions of the upper and lower respiratory tract may decrease in patients with SS, producing dryness of the nose, throat, and trachea; may result in a chronic dry cough. Low secretions of the exocrine glands of the skin could result to dry skin, and vaginal dryness may cause pruritus, irritation, and dyspareunia. Systemic manifestations of SS could affect the lungs, liver, kidneys, vasculature, and blood. A small percentage of SS patients with certain adverse prognostic factors (purpura, low C4 complement levels, and mixed monoclonal cryoglobulinemia) experience high mortality.

Sjögren's disease also increases the risk of cancer of the lymphatic system (most commonly non-Hodgkin lymphoma) discomfort with a light touch.

Blood involvement can result in low red blood cell counts or anemia (sometimes leading to fatigue and shortness of breath), low white cell counts (sometimes leading to frequent infections), and low platelet counts (sometimes leading to bleeding).

Sjögren's Syndrome an Autoimmune Condition

Sjögren's syndrome is a Chronic autoimmune condition which occurs when the immune system attacks the glands that produce moisture in the eyes, mouth, and other parts of the body.

Impact of Sjögren's Syndrome on the Body

Eyes: As a result of less tear production, your eyes feel extremely dry.

Mouth: Main oral manifestations from Sjögren's syndrome may include a high risk of gingivitis, oral candidiasis, caries, and enlargement of the salivary glands among others.

Skin: By far the most common skin conditions associated with Sjögren are xerosis, or clinically dry skin, and eczematous dermatitis.

Nervous System: The CNS manifestations of pSS include diffuse abnormalities (psychiatric changes, encephalopathy, aseptic meningitis, and cognitive difficulties/dementia) and focal or multifocal involvement of the brain and spinal cord.

Kidney: Lupus nephritis occurs when lupus autoantibodies affect structures in your kidneys that filter out waste.

Liver: The hepatic manifestation of sjögren's syndrome includes primary biliary cirrhosis, HCV, non-alcoholic fatty liver disease, and autoimmune hepatitis.

Joint & Muscle: Your joints may be painful and swollen due to inflammation, or you might feel that various parts of your body, such as your muscles, are achy and tender.

Blood Vessels: Vasculitis is an inflammation of the blood vessels, which then become scarred and too narrow for blood to get through to reach the organs.

Pancreas: Notably, the pancreas is an exocrine gland with a similar function and structure to the salivary glands, and some studies suggest that pancreatic dysfunction is common among Sjogren's patients.

The Brain: Most patients experience "brain fog" symptoms, which manifest as memory lapses, forgetfulness, mental confusion, and difficulties in concentrating, organizing, or anticipating future events.

Swollen Salivary Glands: Certain glands become inflamed, which reduces the production of tears and saliva, causing the main symptoms of Sjögren's syndrome, which are dry eyes and dry mouth.

Chapter Three

Sjögren's Syndrome Diagnosis and Treatments

When I had dry eyes and mouth, and I visited the hospital, my doctor used these steps to confirm Sjögren's syndrome:

Steps to a Proper Diagnosis

- **Examination of the Eyes:** What my doctor did was to examine the cornea, the white portion of the eye, for possible dryness.

- **Lip Biopsy:** My doctor removed cells from a salivary gland. The sample he collected goes to the lab checking for signs of inflammation.

- **Health History:** I was asked if I had a pre-existing autoimmune disease, plus dry eyes and mouth, after which my doctor concluded I was having secondary Sjögren's syndrome.

- **Blood Tests:** These tests when conducted, detected specific antibodies in the blood.

- **Imaging tests:** The particular test done here is called, alometry, which measures how much saliva you produce with the use of X-rays that can detect dye injected into salivary glands.

An Overview of Available Treatment Options

Sjögren's syndrome has no cure but the treatment options focus on the identified symptoms.

In a not shell, treatment options for sjögren's syndrome can be divided into three basic categories:

- Treatment of dry eyes, eyelid irritation(blepharitis)

- Treatment of dry mouth, oral yeast infections, and acid reflux.
- Treatment of fatigue and/or vague symptoms of poor concentration and impaired memory (like fibromyalgia).

Treatment of dry eyes: — Most people prefer eye drops, otherwise referred to as (artificial tears) to treat dry eyes. Several solutions are available; a physician can recommend an adequate type based on your level of dryness and fluid production in the eye.

There is a simple procedure known as punctal occlusion. In this procedure, a tiny plug is inserted into the tear ducts by an ophthalmologist the blocking of this duct enables your tears to stay longer in the eye.

Treatment of dry Mouth: Stimulating saliva — simply sucking on sugar-free candy or lozenges or chewing sugar-free gum can stimulate the flow of saliva.

Preventing cavities — you should brush and floss after eating meals and snacks. I prefer an electric toothbrush.

There is available toothpaste designed specifically for people with dry mouth.

Integrative Approaches to Managing Symptoms

If you have been diagnosed with Sjögren's syndrome, you might be quite fortunate. With standard medical tests, it generally takes about six years to come up with a proper diagnosis. Symptoms vary from person to person, and there is a range of problems that may prompt someone on a move from doctor to doctor, trying to cure or manage this condition.

Mostly the early warning signs are dryness, pain, and fatigue. The Classic Sicca symptoms are dry, gritty eyes; dry mouth; dry skin and rashes; dry cough; vaginal dryness; joint or muscle pain; sore tongue or throat; swollen glands; thyroid problems; and overall tiredness and feeling lethargic.

Unfortunately, seeking medical attention frequently for one or two of these symptoms leads patients to go from one specialist to another, each of them may address part of the problem. Without incorporating and attending to the other symptoms, the patient may develop additional complications, such as pneumonia, pancreatitis, and vasculitis. If diagnosed improperly or untreated could lead to further complications, such as severe abdominal pain; swollen lymph nodes; eye sores or pain; jaundice; or persistent cough with coloured phlegm.

Chapter Four

Living with Sjögren's Syndrome

If you are seeking information on Sjögren's syndrome, carefully select the right source.

Join a Sjögren's Syndrome Foundation Support Group to meet other people with Sjögren's syndrome. You will feel better knowing that you are not alone, you will learn more about Sjögren's syndrome from fellow patients and expert speakers, plus you will find new ways to cope with your disease.

Find a doctor who will handle all of your care for Sjögren's syndrome and lead your "medical care team." Usually, this will be a rheumatologist, but a family doctor or general practitioner can also play this role.

Adjusting to Life with Chronic Illness

Chronic illness could be disturbing leading to discomfort and alteration on the pattern of living. But at least it will surely come to an end. As soon as the bone or belly heals, you are going back to normal. That is not so for high blood pressure, heart failure, diabetes, arthritis, Sjögren's syndrome, or other chronic conditions. With no "cure" available, they are lifetime conditions which can be managed with proper care.

You can live with a chronic condition from day to day, and attending to it quickly reduces its severity.

Below are 8 useful steps for coping with a chronic condition.

- **Get a prescription for information.** The more you know about your condition, the better equipped you'll be to understand what's happening and why.

- **Make your doctor a partner in care.** We'd put this one more bluntly: Take responsibility for your care and don't leave everything to your doctor.

- **Build a team.** Doctors don't have all the answers. Seek out the real experts.

- **Invest in yourself.** Find time for exercise and other recreative activities.

- **Make it a family affair.** Talk to your family members about your condition, with the collaboration of everyone, better ways of handling this disease will be gotten.

- **Manage your medications.** Family members should be made aware on the medication you are taking each, how to administer it.

- **Beware of depression.** Always observe your mood and behaviour, you will know when you are going out of the lane.

Toxic Habits to Avoid

- **Alcohol**. Increases your chance of developing dry mouth dryness.

- **Tobacco**. Cigarette smoking will lead to dry mouth, so avoid it.

- **Caffeinated drinks**. These are not recommended.

- **Avoid very hot and spicy foods**. These can aggravate the burning sensation in the mouth.

- **Avoid** dry, sticky and sugary foods.

Coping with Emotional Challenges and Mental Health

It has been observed that different factors influence the personality of someone with Sjögren's syndrome and lead to psychological changes in affected patients.

It is necessary that such psychological changes are ascertained and dealt with as early as possible.

Below are some ways you can adopt to cope with emotional and mental challenges due to Sjögren's syndrome:

Reduced Level of Activities

Do you prefer to rest continuously instead of participating in any kind of activity? If yes, these could be the first signs of depression and must be attended to immediately.

Low Therapy Compliance

If you notice that you are not interested in taking your medications as expected or are indifferent toward them, consult your doctor as soon as possible.

Loss of Work Productivity

If you or someone you know has been diagnosed with sjögren's syndrome, ensure you inform your workplace human resources manager so he/she can take due cognizance and perform any necessary accommodations.

Increased Physical and Emotional Fatigue

Emotional fatigue occurs due to anxiety and depression, leading to a feeling of hopelessness and failure as well as disturbed sleep. Always have a positive thinking towards your health and condition. Avoid any feeling which inter-fairs with your sleep.

Increased Anger (Paranoid)

If you notice that you are getting agitated without cause at both people and things, you should consult your doctor immediately.

Increased Suicidal Tendencies

If you find that you or someone close to you are talking about things such as the futility of life, or acting recklessly in a manner that could put you or them in danger, consult a psychologist immediately.

Alcohol or Sedatives Dependent

You should not smoke or take any substance to make you forget your agony, and you should avoid areas where people are smoking, as this can worsen dryness symptoms.

Getting Support from Family, Friends, and Healthcare Workers

As Sjögren's patient, you are concerned about your health and that of your loved ones; I know you want to learn more about Sjögren's syndrome.

Here are a few things you can do to establish a support network:

- Expand your knowledge about Sjögren's syndrome by visiting trusted sites with information on Sjögren's syndrome, forms, causes, symptoms, diagnosis and treatment.

- Attend a local support group meeting with your family, friends or healthcare provider.

- Invite your friend or loved one on a visit to your physician's appointment.

- Register with the Sjögren's Foundation. I encourage you to visit the Get Involved page to learn more.

Tips for Communicating with Medical Professionals Effectively

Preparation is key to success. Before attending my first visit, I would write out my objectives for that appointment. Unfortunately, many healthcare providers have had little experience with Sjögren's.

Therefore, it is part of my responsibility to update them with information about my illness.

Ask your professional these questions:

- How many patients have you treated with Sjögrens?

- How many years of experience do you have in managing this condition?

- What is the number of patients you have successfully managed?

If a practitioner is not open to learning about Sjögren's, then I know immediately that this relationship isn't a good one. Below are documents I keep handy during a scheduled appointment with my health care provider:

- Copies of my last few lab and test results.

- A typed list of my current medications/supplements with dosages.

Providing my new practitioner with these lists helps expedite my appointment and serves as an indicator that I am serious about taking an actionable role in managing my health.

Chapter Five

Managing Symptoms

At the moment, there is no cure for Sjögren's syndrome, but there exist treatments that help to minimize symptoms.

Understanding Dry Eyes

Dry eye happens when your eyes don't make enough tears to stay wet, or when your tears don't work correctly as a result of the autoimmune condition "Sjögren's syndrome". This can make your eyes feel uncomfortable, and in some cases, it can also cause blurred vision.

Below is a list of dry eyes symptoms:

- Stinging or burning feelings in your eye

- Red eyes

- Sensitivity to light

- Blurry vision

How do I know if I'm at risk of dry eyes?

Anyone can get dry eyes, but you might be more likely to have dry eyes if you:

- Are age 40 or older.

- Are a female.

- Wear contact lenses.

What are the causes of dry eyes?

When your glands refuse to produce enough tears. This means that:

- Inability of the glands to make adequate tears to keep the eyes wet.

- Your tears dry up too fast

- Your tears not flowing out enough to keep your eyes wet.

What is the treatment for dry eye?

Dry eyes are treated according to the root cause of the symptoms.

Below are some of the few treatments for dry eyes:

Over-the-counter eye drops. Dry eyes can be effectively treated with artificial tears.

Prescription medicines. Cyclosporine (Restasis) is a drug prescribed for the treatment of dry eyes. These medicines are good enough to help you make tears.

Lifestyle changes. Ensure you abstain from things that increase your symptoms.

Your eyes will be in good condition if you:

- Try to avoid smoke, wind, and air conditioning

- Wear wraparound sunglasses when you are outside

- Get enough sleep — about 7 to 8 hours a night

Coping with Dry Mouth and Dental Care

Everyone needs saliva to wet and cleanse their mouths and to digest food. Saliva also prevents infection by controlling the activities of bacteria and fungi in the mouth.

What Causes Dry Mouth?

Dry mouth can be caused by:

- **Side effects of certain medical treatments.** Some drugs that we take can lead to dry mouth such as Venlafaxine, Duloxetine, Albuterol, Zolmitriptan among others.

- **Nerve damage.** A dry mouth can be a result of nerve damage to the head and neck area from an injury or surgery.

- **Surgical removal of the salivary glands.**

- **Lifestyle.** Smoking or chewing tobacco can affect how much saliva you make and increase dry mouth.

Symptoms of Dry Mouth?

Common symptoms include:

- A sticky, dry feeling in the mouth

- Frequent thirst

- A dry feeling in the throat

- A dry, red, raw tongue

- Hoarseness, dry nasal passages, sore throat

Why Is Dry Mouth a Problem?

Besides causing the symptoms mentioned above, dry mouth also increases your risk of gingivitis (gum disease), tooth decay, and mouth infections, such as thrush.

Managing Causes of Dry Mouth

If you think your dry mouth is caused by a certain medication you are taking, talk to your doctor. The doctor may adjust the dose you are taking or switch you to a drug that does not cause dry mouth.

But if the medical condition causing the dry mouth can not be changed -- for example, if the salivary gland has been damaged or is a result of disease itself.

Preventing Tooth Decay Due to Dry Mouth

Follow these steps blow to prevent tooth decay and dry mouth:

- Maintain good oral by brushing at least twice a day.

- Flossing your teeth every day

- Use toothpaste that contains fluoride

- Make regular visit to your dentist and optician for a routine check on your mouth and eyes.

Addressing Joint Pain and Fatigue

Joint pain and fatigue do not exist on their own but are symptoms of certain diseases such as flu and Sjögren's syndrome.

Causes of joint pain and fatigue

The following are the causes of sudden joint pain and fatigue:

- Lupus

- Brucellosis

- Rheumatoid arthritis

- Vaccines

- Influenza Virus

- Septic arthritis

Symptoms of Joint Pain and Fatigue

The following are the symptoms of joint pain and fatigue:

- difficulty breathing

- chest pain or pressure

- new confusion

- difficulty staying awake

- severe muscle pain

- severe weakness or loss of balance

- lack of urination

- seizures

Dealing with Skin and Organ-Related Symptoms

One of the notable symptoms of Sjögren's syndrome is dry skin.

Here are steps on caring for your skin if you have sjogren's syndrome.

Visit a Dermatologist

Consult a dermatologist, if you observe any rashes on your skin.

Protect Your Skin against Sunlight

How to protect your skin from sunlight is highlighted below:

Using Mild Soaps on Your Skin

Use soap bar that contain glycerin instead of those that contain fragrances and other chemical ingredients.

Do Not Completely Dry Your Skin

Ensure your skin is not cleaned completely after taking your bath, this will allow moisture on your skin.

Humidifier should be in Dry Environments

A humidifier should be used in environments with dry air. A humidity range between 30% and 50% is ideal for breathing comfortably indoors. However, make sure that you don't raise the humidity level too high, this can encourage the growth of allergens and mould.

Dealing with Organ-Related Symptoms (Nervous System)

When a nervous system is over-reactive you experience symptoms such as:

- Anxiety

- Insomnia

- Panic attacks

- Feelings of hopelessness

- Exhaustion

- Hypertension (high blood pressure)

How to Maintain a Calm Nervous System?

You will not always need prescription pills in order to heal your nervous system. (Although, you are required to consult with your doctor if you are having some symptoms!)

Reset your nervous system with the easy steps below:

- Practice Deep Breathing

Apply Emotional Freedom Technique (EFT)

There are 5 steps you can follow under (EFT):

- Identify your about your condition.

- Set a benchmark level of intensity ranging from 0 to 10.

- Accept who you are with your whole heart.

- Begin to memorize positive events that have happened in the past.

- Assess yourself if you have gotten a 0 level in your worries.

Reduce Your Adrenaline Output Naturally

Have you considered your body may be getting an adrenaline high from intense TV shows and true crime podcasts? Note that, your nervous system does not know the difference between a stressful event happening in real life and those on TV.

The following activities will help you reduce your adrenaline levels:

- Spend more time outdoors

- Identify the primary cause of your condition

- Do some breath work

- Start practicing meditation

- Reduce caffeine intake

- Engage in regular exercise

- Try partaking in yoga

- Perform muscle relaxation techniques.

Chapter Six

Diet and Nutrition

Instead of increasing nutrients and healthy proteins in your diet, the Sjögren's diet lowers or eradicates foods that can cause inflammation or trigger allergic reactions.

Importance of Balanced Diet in Sjögren's Syndrome

The clinician's role should be to support appropriate and evidence-based dietary and supplemental means to reduce systemic inflammation, which may slow disease progression and help reduce symptoms.

It appears that diets focused on reducing inflammation may positively impact symptomatology. While there is no clear evidence on which diet is preferential, it's likely that guiding patients toward more healthful eating patterns that meet their nutritional needs can only help in disease management.

Below is the importance of a Balanced Diet in Sjögren's syndrome

- Eating a balanced diet may help modulate the immune response and thereby improve symptomatology, or even help prevent the condition.

- Anti-inflammatory diets often promote greater omega-3 fatty acid consumption, which results in a more healthful balance with omega-6 and -9 fatty acids.

- Turmeric added to food or taken as a dietary supplement might be helpful in a comprehensive nutrition plan to target inflammation.

Foods that can Alleviate Symptoms

About 90% of people with Sjogren's syndrome have gastrointestinal challenges. Below are some diet preferences used in alleviating Sjogren's syndrome:

Omega-3 fatty acids

This includes foods like fish, nuts, olive oil, and avocados, all of which are anti-inflammatory.

Organic meat

The following meat are good for Sjogren's patients: Beef (Cow), Sheep, Fowls, Grass Cutters, and Rabbits.

Whole fruits and vegetables

The many colourful varieties of fruits and vegetables are loaded with anti-inflammatory nutrients.

Healthy Fruits for Sjögren's Syndrome

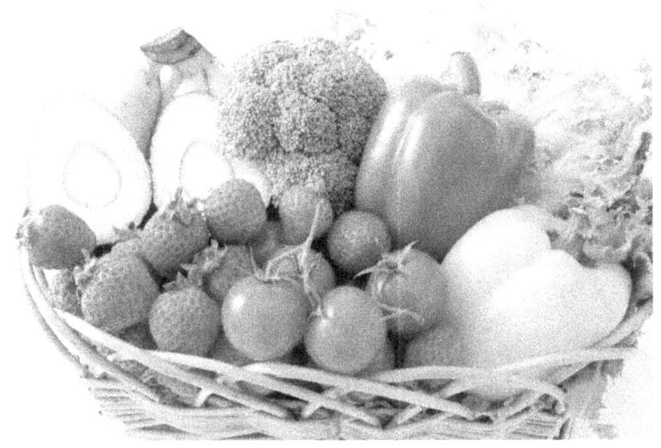

High fibre

Lentils, kidney beans, quinoa, oats, and more are all high-fibre foods that ease symptoms of inflammation.

Spices and herbs

Different seasonings such as garlic or turmeric have long been recognized for their anti-inflammatory benefits.

Specific Nutrients and Supplements that may be beneficial

A series of interventions using specific natural products and Nutrients may provide therapeutic benefits in Sjögren syndrome. **Omega-3 Fatty Acids**

Gamma Linolenic Acid

The omega-6 fatty acid gamma-linolenic acid (GLA) has anti-inflammatory properties.

White Peony Extract

Peony glucosides are biologically active constituents from white peony (*Paeonia*) root, a traditional Chinese medicinal herb.

Lactoferrin

Lactoferrin is an iron-binding protein found in human milk and other body secretions including saliva and tears.

Vitamin D

It has been proven that vitamin D supplements is effective in treating dry eyes and protects against complications arising from Sjogren's syndrome. For autoimmune diseases it is good to take vitamin D at levels of 1,200 to 1,800 IU each day.

N-Acetylcysteine

Reactive oxygen species are eliminated with the help of N-acetylecysteine (NAC), this is because NAC has anti-inflammatory capability. Research has proven that NAC can be used to treat different disease conditions most especially autoimmune diseases.

Maqui Berry Extract (*Aristotelia chilensis*)

Maqui berry (*Aristotelia*) is a tropical berry rich in anthocyanin pigments, which give the berries a dark red or purple colour (Watson 2015). In its native Chile, maqui berry has been used for centuries as a traditional medicine to promote wound healing and improve stamina and strength (Romanucci 2016).

Probiotics

Probiotics has the ability to moderate immune system in inflammatory diseases. An inflammatory disease has a reduced impact on the immune due to the presence of probiotics.

Green Tea Extract

According the New York (Reuters Health) – it states that green tea has a compound which has the ability to lower or better still prevent type 1 diabetes.

A lot of antioxidants are found in green tea which is capable of preventing inflammation, cells death and even cancer.

An extract from green tea can help prevent Sjogren's Syndrome "Medical College of Georgia March, 2007"

Resveratrol

Resveratrol is a plant polyphenol with anti-inflammatory, oxidative stress-reducing, and immune-modulating effects.

Iron, Vitamin B12, and Folic Acid

Iron and vitamin deficiencies frequently occur in individuals with primary sjögren syndrome. Vitamin B12 deficiency in sjögren syndrome results primarily from malabsorption of this vitamin. (Sugaya 1995; Maury 1985).

High homocysteine levels promote neurodegeneration and increase the risk of cardiovascular disease (Stanger 2009; Ganguly 2015). Early detection of these nutrient deficiencies and repletion with appropriate oral supplementation may prevent potentially serious complications and protect the overall health of people with sjögren syndrome (Andres 2001).

Tips for Staying Hydrated and Preventing Malnutrition

About 20% of our daily fluid intake comes from the food we eat and the rest from the liquids we drink.

The amount of water one takes depends on the sex you were assigned at birth.

Tips for staying hydrated

- **Invest in a fun or fancy water bottle.** A good water bottle can serve as a visual reminder to drink more water throughout the day.

- **Focus on your body's signals.** Sometimes we overeat because we mistake thirst for hunger.

- **Drink a glass of water before each meal.**

- **Check the colour of your urine.**

- **Swap high-sugar drinks for sparkling water or seltzer.**

- **Set a daily goal.**

Preventing Malnutrition

Your eating pattern should follow thus:

- Plenty of fruit and vegetables

- Consume much of rice, bread, potatoes, pasta

- Eating some proteins such as meat, eggs, fish, and beans

- Snack between meals

- Have drinks that contain lots of calories

Chapter Seven

Exercise and Physical Activity

There are many types of physical activity, including swimming, running, jogging, walking, and dancing, among others.

As long as it is moderately done, exercise and physical activity reduce chronic inflammation.

Impact of Regular Exercise on Sjogren's Syndrome

1. Exercise can make you feel better

Exercise has been shown to improve your mood and reduce feelings of depression, anxiety, and stress.

3. Exercise can increase your energy levels. Regular physical activity improves your muscle strength and increases your endurance.

4. Exercise can help skin health. With exercise your skin cells are nourished. Oxygen and nutrients are carried to living cells all through the body and the skin by the blood.

5. Exercise can help with relaxation and improve sleep quality. Exercise improves sleep. Exercise also reduces the time people take to fall asleep. It leads to better sleep mood and improved mental health.

7. Exercise can reduce pain. Regular exercise prevents joint pain, muscle tightness and proper blood circulation.

8. Exercise can promote a better sex life

Exercise has been proven to boost sex drive. Exercise can help improve sexual desire, function, and performance in men and women.

Benefits of Regular Physical Activities

Physical activity is important for your overall health. Here, we will look at some of the benefits of regular movement or exercise and what the research shows.

1. Better heart health

For better heart health physical activity:

- strengthening the heart muscle
- helps to control blood pressure and blood fat
- reducing inflammation

2. Lower risk of stroke

Getting enough physical activity may also reduce your chances of having a stroke.

3. Stronger muscles and bones

Exercise helps your muscles grow stronger; they have better effects on the bones. The tougher the exercise the more those bones are strengthened. If you do not engage in regular exercise, your muscles will become very weak over time.

4. More energy

Aerobic exercise is good for improving the levels of energy. There is an increase in heart beat and oxygen usage by the body, this leads to better cardiovascular condition.

6. Better sleep

Exercising for at least 1hour each day especially in the evening could improve your sleep level and promote good quality sleep.

Low-impact Exercise Suitable for Individuals with Joint Pain

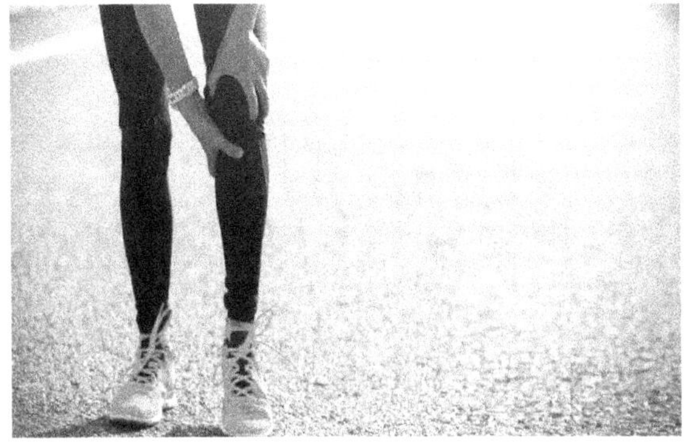

If you suffer from arthritis or joint pain, you may have heard your friends or even your doctor tells you that exercise is a great way to alleviate joint pain. While it is true that some exercises can be painful, especially if you have arthritis, not every exercise has to be so strenuous on your joints. Below are 7 exercises that are great for joint pain,

- **Walking** – If you are not walking, it means you are sitting too much, which can lead to lower back and hip pain.

- **Stretching** – Stretching helps to alleviate muscle pain and tightness, as well as to increase flexibility, movement, and range of motion which, in turn, will help to alleviate joint pain.

- **Core Workouts** - The following exercises are good for improving strength, balance, coordination, and core strength, which will improve your ability to take part in other exercises as well as help alleviate joint pain.

Yoga – Yoga is a low-impact exercise that can help improve coordination, balance, strength, flexibility and range of motion. Yoga combines stretching and body poses with breathing and meditation exercises which help to improve positional body awareness. The combination of muscle strengthening increased flexibility and body awareness help to greatly improve balance.

Increasing Strength, Lowering Impact

People who suffer from rheumatoid arthritis are at increased risk of heart disease and can greatly benefit from aerobic exercises. Below are some exercises with increased cardiovascular intensity that still lower impact on your joints.

- **Water Aerobics** – Water aerobics incorporates many of the high -intensity exercises of a typical aerobics class, but is low impact due to the weight displacement of the water.

- **Cycling** – Pedaling a bike has a much lower impact on the knees and ankles than running or walking, making it a great aerobic and strengthening exercise for the lower body.

Strength Training

One of the key aspects of all the aerobic exercises listed above is that they all offer strength training exercises as well. As you strengthen your muscles, it puts less strain on the joints.

Weight-Bearing Exercises: – Weight-bearing exercises includes exercise that builds muscle using free weights, machines, or resistance bands.

Benefits of Low-Impact Exercise Suitable for Individuals with Joint Pain

Low-impact exercises help stress low joints while you move. Examples include stationary or recumbent bicycling, elliptical trainer workouts, or exercise in the water.

Creating an exercise routine tailored to individual needs and limitations

If you're considering starting to exercise but don't know where to begin, this book is for you. Here's all you need to know about starting a routine and staying within your limit.

Why exercise?

Regular exercise can help improve mental function, reduce your risk for chronic disease and manage your weight.

Common types of exercise

There are various types of exercise, including: swimming, running, dancing, cardio machines, walking, hiking, cross-country skiing, and kickboxing.

Chapter Eight

Sleep and Fatigue Management

Insomnia is the inability to feel sleepy at night hours. This lack of sleep can be frustrating and impact your day-to-day living and quality of life.

Understanding the Relationship between Sjögren Syndrome and Fatigue

I have come up with the following sub-types of fatigue your experience may be different:

- **Basic fatigue:** Those with this fatigue find it difficult to get out of bed in the morning and this stops someone from meeting up with their daily routine activities.

- **Sudden fatigue:** It comes on suddenly, and I have to stop whatever I'm doing and just sit down (as soon as I can).

- **Molten lead phenomenon:** It feels as if someone has poured molten lead into my head and on all my limbs while I slept. My muscles and joints hurt and doing anything is like walking with heavy weights.

- **Fatigue related to other physical causes:** Fatigue related to other physical causes, such as thyroid problems or anemia or other diseases superimposed on Sjögren's.

- **Fatigue that comes from a chronic illness that just won't quit:** There is fatigue that comes with the uncertainty of a chronic disease.

Strategies for improving sleep quality and managing daytime fatigue

The effect of long-term sleep deprivation can be far more serious, increasing the risk of coronary heart disease, stroke, diabetes, obesity and Alzheimer's disease. Below are 7 tops ways of improving sleep quality:

Top 10 Ways to Improving Sleep Quality

1. Have time for relaxation

Make sure you create enough time for relaxation each day, it will help improve the quality of your sleep.

2. Create a restful environment

Ensure your resting place is comfortable for you including your bed.

3. Foods for sleeping

Eating milk, chicken, turkey and pumpkin seeds can greatly improve your sleep.

4. Foods to avoid

Avoid spicy foods and alcohol entirely.

5. Darkness promotes sleep

Before going to bed ensure the lights are turned off, this is because darkness promotes sleep a lot.

6. Avoid late night consumption of Caffeine

When caffeine is taken late at night, your nervous system is activated and this could lead to inability to have a relaxation at night.

7. Reduce your day time naps

Taking a little nap during the day is good for your health, whereas long napping in the day time could affect your sleep. By sleeping in the day time, your body may think that you have completed your sleep for day thereby leading to difficulty in sleeping.

8. Sleeping and waking up at consistent time each day

Consistency with your sleep schedules and getting up can help improve your sleep quality.

9. Going for a melatonin supplement

Melatonin a sleep hormone will tell your brain the due time for relaxation and sleep each day.

10. Do not Take Alcohol

A couple of drinks at night will affect your hormones and sleep.

Managing Daytime Fatigue

The following steps will aid you in managing your daytime sleep.

- **Eat often to beat tiredness**

- **Get moving**

- **Getting enough sleep**

- **Reduce stress to boost energy**

- **Cut out caffeine**

- **Drink less alcohol**

- **Drink more water for better energy**

Creating a Sleep-friendly Environment and Bedtime Routine

Creating a sleep routine that works for you helps you get the needed amount of sleep each night. When creating your bedtime routine, consider the following:

Setting up a sleep-friendly environment - ensure the bedroom is comfortable and relaxing

- Minimize the noise level and make the room dark and cool

- Remove TVs and computer sets from the bedroom

Maintain a consistent sleep schedule—use the same bedtime routine on both weekdays and weekends

- Create a bedtime routine (shower, pyjamas, and brush teeth)

- Set a time to remind you when to go to bed each day.

Chapter Nine

Building Resilience and Self-Care

Resilience is the ability to adapt well in the face of adversity, such as when you may be experiencing personal or family issues, a serious health condition, work stress, lack of money, or other difficulties. It is the ability to recover from challenges.

- **Promoting Self-care Practices to Reduce Stress and Improve Well-being**

- **Pay attention to your physical self-care**

- **Make exercise a routine.**

- **Choose a healthy diet.**

Change your attitude on how you view problems and challenges

See stressful events as opportunities to learn and grow.

Building your emotional resilience to overcome your challenges

Think about other people you know and admire those who are resilient, whether they are public figures or people you may know in your personal or work life.

Keep it simple

Simplifying your life is most important during stressful times.

Make your routines simple and set limits to protect your time. Plan simple meals. Resist engaging in too many activities or over-committing yourself.

Practice relaxation techniques

Deep breathing, meditation, mindfulness, and yoga are four widely used relaxation techniques that can help improve mental and physical well-being.

Techniques for Managing Stress and Anxiety Related to Sjögren Syndrome

Sjogren's syndrome can be stressful and scary to deal with, which is why many tend to be anxious about managing this condition. Here are some techniques you might apply.

Understanding your symptoms
Maintain a positive lifestyle throughout

You should always maintain fit and active lifestyle. Create a plan for managing your leisure and work.

Avoid anything that triggers your symptoms

Autoimmune diseases such as Sjogren's syndrome are likely to be triggered by environmental factors such as pollution, infections, certain medications, diet, and allergens.

Try to relax

Proper relaxation will relieve you of anxiety and depression all the time.

Mindfulness and Meditation Exercise to Cope with Chronic Illnesses

Chronic illness can take many different forms, but the feelings that usually come with it are almost the same — anxiety, confusion, depression, and stress.

When I tell people that meditation helped me cope with chronic illness, they often seem doubtful. But in my own life and for the diabetic patient I worked with, I have found that meditation can be a powerful coping and healing tool.

The power of mindfulness

Human beings are always doing this, most of the time without being aware or mindful. We go through our day, doing. Always doing. Rarely ever just being.

But especially when you have a chronic illness, it's important to take a few minutes to just be calm and reflect.

Applying meditation

I'm hoping that you will use these guidelines to practice mediation on your own time:

- Remain focused. A simple acknowledgement and re-focusing on the breath is all it takes to redirect your meditation.

- Be quiet. Keep breathing. Remember to breathe with purpose, practice and repetition.

- Be present. If negative thoughts appear, they should be identified and discarded, like clouds floating across a blue sky.

- Even a few moments of focused breathing and mindfulness can help you relax, which is important in managing all types of stress. The more you practice meditation, the stronger you will become, both mentally and physically.

Your chronic illness does not have to change who you are. Take a few moments and try practicing meditation today.

Chapter Ten

Work, Education, and Social Life

It took me four long years to receive my sjögren's diagnosis.

As soon as I received my diagnosis, I was relieved, but I also knew life would not go back to being normal—ever. Yes, I received treatment, which helped, but fatigue and pain are constant. I deal with them daily.

Navigating Work or Educational Environment while Managing Symptoms

The fact that I had this condition does not prompt me to withdraw from work, education or social activities, but I developed mechanisms to navigate through life and still maintain my relationship with friends, colleagues and family members in the following ways:

- Working from home, which allows me to rest as required.

- Educating people about my disease. I give out leaflets to people in a bid to educate them about this condition.

- Carefully planning my schedule. If I plan to go to a concert on a Friday, I know I will need the entire weekend to recover and rest.

Requesting accommodations and understanding legal rights

According to the Job Accommodation Network, there is no exhaustive list of accommodations that must be provided under the Americans with Disabilities Act. While all autoimmune diseases and symptoms are different, this is a substantial list of reasonable accommodations so you can begin with.

- Allow for flexible work and leave schedule.

- Allow periodic and/or longer breaks.

- Reduce job stress.

- Reduce or eliminate physical exertion.

- Provide parking close to the worksite.

- Switch to an ergonomic chair.

- Keep the work environment free from dust, smoke, odour and fumes.

- Redirect air conditioning and heating vents.

- Provide sensitivity training to coworkers.

- Provide information on counseling and employee assistance programs.

Maintaining an Active Social Life and Managing Social Interactions

You can start improving your social skills by following these 5 strategies and soon, you will be able to enter into conversations with confidence.

1. Act like a Social Person

2. Start Small if Necessary

3. Encourage Others to Talk about Themselves

4. Read Books about Social Skills

5. Join a Social Skills Support Group

Chapter Eleven

Travelling and Sjogren Syndrome

Tips for Safe and Enjoyable Travel with Sjogren Syndrome

- Arrive early at the airport

- Follow TSA guidelines

TSA Guidelines for Air Travel by Sjogren's Patients

Planning for Medical Needs While Away from Home

Before you embark on your trip, make a plan for how you will get health care when travelling.

- Get travel insurance.

- Take recommended medicines as directed.

Chapter Twelve

Pregnancy and Family

Will being pregnant make my sjögren's worse? Special Considerations for Women with Sjogren's Syndrome During Pregnancy.

Consideration for Conception

You should discuss family planning issues with your rheumatologist early on, not just when you have decided you would like to start having a baby, according to Dr. Sammaritano. While there's a possibility that your child may develop Sjögren's or another autoimmune disease, it's important to remember that many women with autoimmune diseases have healthy babies who don't have Sjögren's or other autoimmune disease.

Effect of pregnancy on Sjogren's: For many women, sjögren's worsens during pregnancy and/or after delivery. This makes it important to not only see your rheumatologist regularly but to also plan for extra help after the baby arrives.

Consideration during Pregnancy

If the drugs you were taking at conception are controlling your disease, your doctor will likely have you continue with them throughout pregnancy, provided they are compatible with pregnancy. **Effects on delivery.** While most women with sjögren's can deliver vaginally, any complications with you or the baby could necessitate an early delivery by C-section.

Consideration During Breastfeeding

For most women with sjögren's, a healthy delivery and baby is possible. **Disease activity:** If you notice worsening symptoms, contact your rheumatologist, because some women experience increased disease activity after delivery.

Medication and breastfeeding: If controlling your disease after delivery requires a change in medication, be sure to let your doctor know if you are breastfeeding.

Family Planning Options and Considerations

Easy Contraception to Apply:

The most effective birth control method for "real world" use is the one that is simplest for you.

Chapter Thirteen

Future Research and Hope

This disease predominantly affects women, with an estimated female-to- male ratio of 14 to 1.

The discovery of pSS-associated loci

In pSS, four GWAS, one large-scale study employing the Immuno-Chip (a custom SNP array) and other large-scale arrays, a targeted sequencing study of five candidate's genes shows different loci of genome-wide which is predominant in European populations.

Sex Hormones

Differential immunomodulatory effects elicited by sex hormones have obvious potential to contribute to the sex bias in pSS, however, studies on sex hormone levels in patients with pSS are remarkably limited, and the results are inconsistent.

X chromosome Gene Dosage

Although no SNP associations with pSS have yet been identified on this chromosome, the importance of the X chromosome in pSS is supported by studies of aneuploidy. The frequency of aneuploidy in patients with pSS is low, but several studies support an X chromosome dosage effect on the risk of pSS.

Targeting DNA Methylation

Modification of DNA methylation is a potential therapeutic intervention for various diseases, as exemplified by the successful employment of such drugs in the field of immuno-oncology. Available drugs that modify DNA methylation are employed for the treatment of various cancers. However, these drugs, including azacytidine and decitabine, are DNA methyltransferase inhibitors, and they function in a nonspecific manner to reduce genomic DNA methylation, which could be counterproductive for the treatment of pSS, given that pSS-associated genes tend to be hypomethylated. Indeed, the drugs hydralazine and procainamide, which inhibit DNA methylation, have long been known to confer a high risk of triggering drug-induced SLE.

Encouragement and hope for individuals living with Sjögren's Syndrome

Sjögren's Syndrome (SJS) diagnosis and classification remains a challenge, especially at the initial stage of the condition, when patients may have milder phenotypes of the disease or uncommon presentations.

Worldwide, several drugs are being tested in small, randomized trials in the hopes that they may produce targeted treatment for specific manifestations of the disease. A clinician and researcher, St. Clair is working tirelessly with patients who have Sjögren's syndrome and investigations are ongoing into new treatment areas.

Inspiring Stories of Resilience and Success

The Farmer and the Donkey

One day a farmer's donkey fell down into a well.

He invited all of his neighbours to come over and help him. Then, to everyone's amazement, he quieted down.

He was astonished at what he saw.

As the farmer's neighbours continued to shovel dirt on top of the animal, he would shake it off and take a step up.

Life is going to shovel dirt on you, all kinds of dirt including chronic illnesses. The trick to getting out of the well of anxiety and depression is to shake it off and take a step up.

Personal disability story: – Therese's story.

Therese's story

Therese with her daughter

I have a connective tissue disease called Sjogren's syndrome and have recently been told I may also have Lupus. I also have Myoclonic seizures on an almost daily basis. These have to be controlled by a raft of medications, so the flexibility of working from home allows me to deal with the side effects of the medication such as extreme fatigue.

Chapter Fourteen

Resources and Support

Those living with Sjogren's syndrome have opportunity to connect and by sharing their experiences, tips, and suggestions solutions will be gotten on how best to manage this condition.

These groups provide:

- Guided topic discussions related to Sjögren's

- Patient-to-patient sharing of experiences

- Techniques on coping with Sjogren

- Knowledge of helpful resources

List of reputable organizations for Sjogren syndrome

Dedicated caring volunteer members run the Support Groups. Contact the support group leader in your area (by phone or e-mail) to learn more about upcoming meetings.

Below is the list of reputable support groups:

- Sjogren's Society of Canada (SSC)

- The Sjogrens International Collaborative Clinical Alliance (SICCA)

- The British Sjogren Syndrome Association (BSSA)

- The Sjögren's syndrome Philadelphia-area support group is based at Penn Medicine University City (SSPSG)

Websites links for Sjogren Syndrome

- **Website: https://www.sjogrens.org**

- **Website: https://www.pennmedicine.org> sjogrens-syndrome**

- **Website: https://journals.lww.com/ijru/Fulltext/2023/ 1/08**

- **Website:**

  https://www.cambridge.org/core/journals/article

- **Website:**

  https://www.verywellhealth.com/secondary-sjogren

Recommended Books, Articles and Additional Reading Materials for Sjogrens' Syndrome

- Oxford Text of Sjögren's Syndrome: The Oxford Textbook of Sjögren's syndrome is an authoritative textbook, with rich valuable illustrations and figures, providing a practical guide to diagnosing and managing all aspects of this condition.

- Better Choices for Sjogren's Patients: Complete Guide to Coping and Managing the Condition. This book, written by a woman who has Sjögren's Syndrome, presents and evaluates a full range of treatment options……….possible benefits and side-effects.

Conclusion

Sjogren's syndrome is an autoimmune disease that mainly affects the eyes and salivary glands, but can also affect other parts of the body.

It is an autoimmune disease because the immune system attacks the lachrymal and salivary glands causing eyes and mouth dryness.

The exact cause of this condition is not known at the moment. But studies suggest that your gene, virus, bacteria, and triggers may play a role.

The primary symptoms of this disease are dry eyes with burning, irritation, and dry mouth with difficulty swallowing or chewing things.

The disease can be diagnosed through blood tests, biopsies, eye examinations, questioning, and x-ray among others.

Just as the actual cause of this disease is unknown so also the treatment. But treatment focuses on the symptoms.

There are things you can do to manage these conditions yourself, this ranges from sipping water regularly, engaging in regular exercise and physical activities, practicing good oral hygiene, eating moist foods, avoiding salty, acidic or spicy foods and carbonated drinks, increasing hydration and avoid dry environment.

There are support groups willing to assist when needed and books, articles and websites to help you manage your conditions for a better life and longevity.

The trauma of living with this disease alone is so depressing and its associated pains and anxiety. It is for sure that the quality of life is affected and coping will be difficult for anyone. It's a wonder that most women with chronic illnesses manage to get out of bed every day, let alone do it with a smile, determination, and grit to keep pushing not minding the numerous obstacles they encounter on daily basis.

It is true majority of those affected by this condition are women, those who have developed ability to cope and manage this illness could be referred to as (Super Women). But what the strongest women need now is inspiration and motivation every now and then to get through those trying moments. With determination can overcome all these troubles and live a healthy life.

Treatment of this condition is mainly focused on the symptoms and not the disease itself because at present there is no known cure for Sjogren's Syndrome. Studying other similar autoimmune diseases will help you understand this condition better, although the 2019 management recommendations from EULAR are now being used to inform clinical management of pSS.

Worldwide, several drugs are being tested in small, randomized trials in the hopes that they may produce targeted treatment for specific manifestations of the disease.